13. Remove excess furniture, equipment, and personnel from area.

14. Support family and visitors. Escort them from the area, if possible, and tell them to remain in a specific area. You will need to locate them later. Provide emotional support. If necessary, refer them to another nurse or a chaplain, social worker, or patient representative.

15. Assure care for other patients on unit. Remove patients from the immediate area or screen them from activities. Assign someone to support and provide care for the patients in unit.

16. Notify attending doctor. Ask resuscitation team leader (if any) if he prefers to speak to the attending doctor.

17. Provide necessary equipment from floor stock.

18. Complete resuscitation effort. If successful, transfer patient to monitored area, observe recurrent arrhythmias, and arrange for the doctor to speak with the family. If unsuccessful, be sure doctor has notified the family and completed autopsy consent forms, if requested; perform postmortem care and provide emotional support for the family. Check and restock resuscitation equipment. Arrange for backup equipment during restocking.

THE NURSE'S REFERENCE LIBRARY®

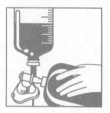

Procedures

Nursing83 Books™
Intermed Communications, Inc.
Springhouse, Pa.

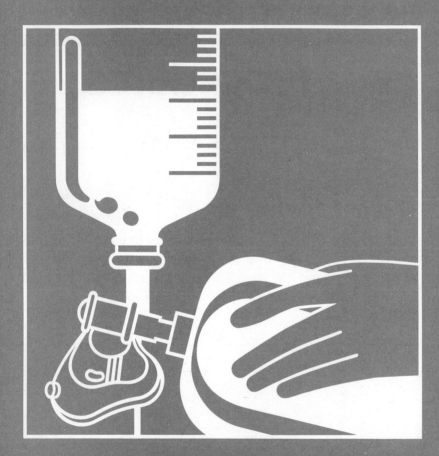